Mastering Metformin

*Your Essential Guide
to Diabetes Control*

Christopher Garland

Copyright@ 2024

This book is a work of nonfiction. While every effort has been made to ensure accuracy, the author and publisher assume no responsibility for errors or omissions.

The information provided in this guidebook is for educational purposes and does not constitute medical advice. Always consult a health care professional before starting or changing any medical treatment.

Table of Contents

Chapter One

Introduction

For the millions of people suffering from diabetes, imagine finding a key that would open the door to a better, more balanced life.

Metformin is a symbol of this. However many people find the term "Type 2 diabetes" overwhelming and alienating. It's a lifeline that has enabled innumerable people to take charge of their health rather than just a tablet.

Biguanides are a class of medications that includes the pharmaceutical metformin. For those with Type 2 diabetes, its main goal is to reduce blood sugar levels.

Metformin lets people live full, active lives without having to constantly worry about their blood sugar levels being out of control. But it does more than that. It helps people manage their illness.

Eventually, in the 1950s, metformin was presented to the medical community, and its ability to control blood sugar levels won praise before long. At its foundation, metformin functions by assisting the body in controlling glucose, the chemical that powers our cells.

An individual's body has trouble using insulin as intended when they have Type 2 diabetes. One hormone called insulin makes it possible for glucose to enter cells and be used as fuel.

A malfunction of this system causes glucose to accumulate in the blood, which can eventually result in high blood sugar levels and major problems. When metformin is taken, the body becomes more sensitive to insulin and the liver produces less glucose.

Your blood sugar levels will drop to healthier ranges as a result of your body being able to utilise the insulin it already has more efficiently. Helping your body discover balance and stability is akin to gently nudging it in the right way.

Yet the effects of metformin go beyond managing blood sugar. As a typical consequence of diabetes, heart disease, studies have shown that it can also lower the risk of heart disease.

For a lot of people, metformin offers a chance to enhance general health and well being in addition to helping them control their diabetes.

Metformin is quite safe, very effective, and well-tolerated by most people, as evidenced by numerous studies. Because it provides a gradual introduction to managing the condition, it is frequently the first medicine offered to patients who have just received a Type 2 diabetes diagnosis.

Metformin is a consistent and dependable option because, in contrast to some diabetes drugs, it doesn't produce sharp fluctuations in blood sugar.

Moreover, weight increase is usually not a problem for those who have diabetes. To help with the condition's management, some people may even find that metformin encourages weight loss.

Chapter Two

The Role of Metformin in Diabetes Management

For people suffering from Type 2 diabetes, metformin acts as a quiet protector. It does its best job of assisting your body in controlling blood sugar levels while operating silently in the background.

Metformin helps prevent those hazardous blood sugar surges that can seriously damage your health by lowering the quantity of glucose your liver produces and enhancing your body's response to insulin.

If the body either stops producing insulin or develops an intolerance to it, type 2 diabetes will result. Glucose, or sugar, can enter your cells and deliver energy like a key that opens their doors thanks to insulin.

Blood glucose levels rise as a result of insulin's inability to function properly. If untreated over time, this might lead to major side effects such kidney failure, nerve damage, heart disease, and visual issues.

Regulating Blood Sugar

Most people associate metformin with being a treatment for diabetes. The narrative, however, goes beyond only controlling blood sugar, metformin has several other advantages.

It is an even more important component of managing diabetes because research has revealed that it has several extra beneficial benefits on the body.

Its advantageous effects on heart health are among the most notable. Although metformin can help reduce the risk of heart disease, those with diabetes are still far more likely to get it.

It's an essential component of a holistic approach to diabetes care because studies have shown that it lowers the risk of heart attacks and strokes. It has been discovered that metformin helps with weight management in addition to heart protection.

Managing Type 2 diabetes can be made more difficult by the fact that many individuals with the disease struggle with weight gain.

Those who take Metformin find that the medication becomes a routine part of their life, providing steadiness in an otherwise uncertain world. It serves as a reminder that despite their situation, people are not helpless and are actively taking care of their health.

Although millions of people worldwide still start with metformin, others may require additional drugs or insulin to completely control their blood sugar. Health care practitioners always turn to it because of its broad range of benefits, ease of use, and efficacy.

Chapter Three

Dosage & Administration

Metformin is one of the safest and most successful first-line therapies for Type 2 diabetes, which is why your health care professional has carefully selected it, They take great care in making this choice.

Probably prior to writing a prescription for Metformin, your physician evaluated your general health, your current blood sugar readings (including A1C), and whether or not diet and exercise adjustments have been sufficient to manage your diabetes.

The next natural step is to take metformin if it's evident that your body needs a little extra support. In most cases, your doctor will put you on a low dose of metformin and increase it gradually as your body becomes used to it.

Giving your body more time to adjust to the drug and reducing side effects are the two main goals of this.

Most people start off taking 500 mg once daily, but depending on your particular needs, your doctor may gradually increase the amount to 1,000 mg or more.

Immediate-release and extended-release tablets are the two types of metformin available. For the purpose of minimizing adverse effects related to digestion, the extended-release form should normally be taken once daily, whereas the immediate-release form should be taken two to three times a day with meals.

Based on factors like your lifestyle, tolerance, and how well the medication affects your blood sugar, your doctor will choose which type is best for you.

To help prevent some of the more uncomfortable side effects related to the digestive system, which we will talk about shortly, it is important to take Metformin with food. In addition to lowering your chance of stomach distress, meals facilitate your body's easier absorption of the drug.

Never forget that the goal is to establish a regimen that benefits both your health and your life, not merely to take a pill.

Chapter Four

Metformin Side Effects

When taking Metformin on a daily basis, millions of people have minor to rare adverse effects. Recognizing potential hazards, developing coping strategies, and knowing when to seek assistance are the most important things.

Metformin may have a unique set of side effects, though, just like any medicine. Realize that you're not the only one going through this.

Knowing the possible side effects, both frequent and uncommon, is crucial. Your ability to handle discomfort, take initiative, and recognize when to seek medical assistance is enhanced by this information.

Minor Side Effects

Digestion-related side effects are the most frequent ones caused by metformin, and although they might be unpleasant, they are usually temporary and easy to handle:

- Gastrointestinal (GI) Issues
- Nausea
- Diarrhea
- Bloating and Gas
- Stomach Cramps

Handling Less Common Side Effects

There are a few less frequent adverse effects that are nevertheless noteworthy to highlight, even if gastrointestinal problems are the most regular ones.

If you are aware of these, you will be more equipped to handle situations when they come up.

Low Level of Vitamin B12

Vitamin B12 insufficiency is one possible long-term adverse effect of metformin. The vital vitamin that is needed for nerve function and the synthesis of red blood cells may not be absorbed by your body as well if you are taking metformin.

Fatigue, weakness, memory issues, and even tingling or numbness in your hands and feet might develop over time as a result of this deficiency.

B12 insufficiency is fortunately easily treated. Especially if you have been taking Metformin for a number of years, your doctor would probably periodically check your B12 levels. Should they find that you are deficient in B12, doctors can suggest B12 shots or pills.

Metallic Taste

When starting Metformin, some patients have a metallic aftertaste in their mouth. It may irritate you, even though it's harmless. After several days or weeks, this flavor normally disappears. Chewing gum or sugar-free candies are good options to numb the flavor in the interim.

Major Side Effects

Although "lactic acidosis" is an uncommon but dangerous side effect to be cautious of, the majority of Metformin users only suffer moderate side effects.

When the bloodstream accumulates lactic acid more quickly than it can be eliminated, the condition is known as lactic acidosis.

Although very unusual, especially in those without a history of renal or liver problems, it is potentially fatal. The following are some of the signs of lactic acidosis:

- ☐ Extreme tiredness or weakness
- ☐ Trouble breathing
- ☐ Unusual muscle pain
- ☐ Sudden dizziness or feeling lightheaded
- ☐ Slowed or irregular heartbeat
- ☐ Feeling cold, particularly in your hands and feet

- ● ☐Stomach pain or discomfort

Make sure you get medical help right away if you have any of these symptoms, especially if they appear unexpectedly.

It is important to treat these symptoms seriously even though there is a low chance of lactic acidosis.

When to Get in Touch with Your Physician

Knowing when to seek medical assistance for side effects is crucial. Metformin's adverse effects are often tolerable and get better with time, but in certain cases, you should contact your doctor right away.

Call your doctor if

1. The symptoms you're experiencing related to your stomach are severe or persist for several weeks.

2. Your hands or feet may tingle, you may feel weak, or you may be experiencing signs of a vitamin B12 shortage.

3. You become aware of the signs of lactic acidosis, such as weakness, dyspnea, chest discomfort, etc.

4. You encounter any unusual-seeming adverse effects or ones that are really uncomfortable.

Your doctor is there to help you through these challenges. Never hesitate to reach out if you're unsure about a side effect or if something doesn't feel right. It's better to ask questions and get reassurance than to worry in silence.

Chapter Five

Individuals who can't take Metformin

Often regarded as the best medicine for treating Type 2 diabetes, metformin is a commonly prescribed drug. Metformin may, however, not work the same way for everyone, and different people may experience its side effects and effectiveness in various ways.

In order to make educated decisions about your health and investigate potentially more appropriate alternative therapies, it is critical to understand the reasons why some people may not be able to take metformin.

If you discover that Metformin isn't a good fit for you, it's crucial to keep in mind that you still have other options. You can successfully manage your diabetes with the help of a number of additional drugs and way of life changes.

Older Adults

The processing of drugs such as Metformin may be impacted by the changes our bodies undergo as we age.

Sustaining independence and quality of life while avoiding complications is typically a tricky balance in the management of diabetes in older persons.

Though there are certain distinct issues associated with aging, metformin is still a reliable alternative for older persons.

As metformin successfully lowers blood sugar without causing considerable weight gain or increasing the risk of hypoglycemia (low blood sugar), which other drugs may induce, it is often the first-line treatment for Type 2 diabetes in older persons.

Most seniors can safely choose it because it is normally well-tolerated.

Kidney function: is a crucial factor to consider while using metformin in the elderly. Given that metformin is metabolized by the kidneys, it is imperative to constantly monitor kidney health as we age because renal function might deteriorate.

For the continued safety of Metformin, your doctor will perform blood tests to monitor your kidney function on a frequent basis.

Should renal function decline, your physician might modify your dosage or look into other options.

lower Risk of Cardiovascular Complications: Heart disease is more common in older persons with Type 2 diabetes. Because it lowers the risk of heart attacks and strokes, metformin has a number of important heart-protective benefits.

For older persons who are worried about their cardiovascular health, this makes it an extremely useful tool for treating diabetes.

Adolescents and Children

Medications such as Metformin have become essential components of pediatric therapy due to the increasing prevalence of type 2 diabetes in children and adolescents.

Healthy growth and development are the main objectives for younger patients, in addition to blood sugar control. Like it does for adults, metformin helps kids and teenagers by lowering the amount of glucose the liver produces and increasing their sensitivity to insulin.

Maintaining stable blood sugar levels is essential for promoting growth and avoiding issues in children and adolescents.

Metformin for Women with PCOS

Although many people are familiar with Metformin's usage in the treatment of Type 2 diabetes, it is also used to treat PCOS, a hormonal condition that affects a large number of women who are of reproductive age. Insulin resistance-related symptoms such as irregular periods and infertility can be brought on by PCOS.

Inconsistent menstrual periods, weight gain, and trouble ovulating can all be caused by women with PCOS, who frequently have elevated insulin levels.

Insulin sensitivity is increased and insulin levels are decreased with metformin, which is helpful. Thus, women who are attempting to conceive may have a higher chance of pregnancy as a result of regularized menstrual cycles and more frequent ovulation.

Controlling weight can be quite difficult for a lot of women with PCOS. The management of PCOS symptoms may depend on Metformin's ability to assist weight loss or, at the very least, stop future weight gain. In addition to this benefit, women with PCOS are at a higher risk of acquiring Type 2 diabetes.

Pregnant and Breastfeeding Mothers

Metformin is being utilized more often to help manage diabetes during pregnancy, which is important for the mother and the unborn child.

Notably, metformin is frequently prescribed to control blood sugar during pregnancy, especially for women who have gestational diabetes.

However, the medication should always be used under the direct supervision of a health care professional.

Gestational diabetes, a kind of the disease that affects how the body handles glucose, can be treated with metformin.

The fact that metformin is usually regarded as safe for both mother and child makes it a popular prescription drug for blood sugar control during pregnancy.

Metformin lowers the production of glucose and improves insulin sensitivity, which helps avoid issues including high birth weight, premature delivery, and the chance of developing Type 2 diabetes in the future. **Pregnancy and Metformin Use:** If you were taking Metformin prior to becoming pregnant, your doctor will determine if it's safe for you to continue, especially if you have PCOS or Type 2 diabetes.

Metformin is often continued in the treatment plan during pregnancy since it regulates blood sugar levels without appreciably increasing the risk of hypoglycemia.

Given that very little of the medication enters breast milk, metformin is thought to be safe to take while nursing.

But, in order to make sure that you and your child are safe, it's crucial to talk to your doctor about any concerns you may have.

For your own health, controlling your blood sugar levels after giving birth is crucial, and metformin can help you do so while still enabling you to breastfeed.

Handling Other Conditions with Metformin

Managing one's diabetes is only one aspect of life for certain individuals. Many people manage other medical issues, such as obesity, renal disease, or heart disease, in addition to taking metformin.

Metformin and Heart Health: The heart is shielded from harm by metformin, which is one of its main advantages. The medication metformin can help lower the risk of heart disease in people with diabetes.

Metformin is a beneficial choice for individuals managing diabetes and cardiovascular issues because it lowers blood sugar and raises cholesterol levels, both of which boost heart health.

Metformin and Kidney Health: The majority of people can safely use metformin, however those who have decreased kidney function should exercise caution.

As metformin is metabolized by the kidneys, patients with severe renal impairment might require a different medication or a lower dosage.

To guarantee that metformin stays a safe and useful treatment, regular evaluation of renal function is necessary.

Excessive Alcohol Consumption

Metformin users who drink excessive amounts of alcohol may be more susceptible to lactic acidosis. This is due to the fact that alcohol interferes with the liver's capacity to metabolize lactic acid, and when paired with metformin.

it can significantly increase the risk of lactic acid accumulation in the blood. Moderate alcohol intake is typically seen as safe when taking metformin, with one drink for women and two for men per day.

Metformin might not be the ideal choice for you, though, if you binge drink or drink alcohol excessively.

Your physician can suggest an alternate prescription to prevent the elevated risk of lactic acidosis if alcohol consumption plays a major role in your life and cutting back is not practical.

Regardless, establishing a treatment plan that suits your requirements and lifestyle requires honest discussion between you and your health care professional.

Individuals with Severe Dehydration

Lethargy raises the possibility of developing lactic acidosis and can worsen Metformin adverse effects. Metformin may accumulate in the body when the kidneys are unable to properly digest and excrete it due to dehydration.

A person's risk of problems when taking metformin is increased if they are excessively dehydrated, either from illness, excessive heat, or not drinking enough water.

Prior to starting Metformin again, make sure you are properly hydrated and speak with your doctor if you have a high temperature, vomiting, or diarrhea. Drinking lots of water can help lower the risk of moderate dehydration.

On the other hand, in cases of severe or chronic dehydration, your physician might suggest stopping Metformin until your hydration levels stabilize, or they might suggest switching to a less risky medicine in these circumstances.

Individuals with Allergic Reactions to Metformin

A metformin allergic reaction is rare, although it can happen to certain people. A reaction to an allergy might manifest as:

- Rash
- Itching
- Swelling (especially in the face or throat)
- Severe dizziness
- Difficulty in breathing

It is crucial to stop taking Metformin and get medical help right away if you have any of these symptoms.

Chapter Six

Precautions

When used as prescribed, metformin can be a very successful way to manage your diabetes, but as with any medicine, there are some safety and usage guidelines that must be followed.

You can minimize side effects and maximize the benefits of Metformin by following the recommended dosage instructions, keeping an eye out for any dangers, and modifying your lifestyle as needed.

Making sure you closely follow your doctor's recommendations is the most crucial safety measure when taking Metformin.

As easy as it may seem, following the dosage and time guidelines can have a significant impact on the medication's effectiveness and your body's ability to handle it.

Stabilizing your blood sugar levels and lowering your risk of gastrointestinal side effects like nausea or diarrhea can be achieved by taking Metformin at the same time every day, ideally with a meal.

When using immediate-release metformin, it may be necessary to take it two or three times a day with meals, but extended-release formulations are usually taken once daily.

Missed Dosage

It is possible for side effects or blood sugar swings to result from missing doses or taking excessive amounts of Metformin.

Until it's almost time for your next scheduled dose, take the missed dose as soon as you recall. Then proceed as usual, skipping the missed dose. To make up for a missed dose, never take two of the same.

Chapter Seven

Metformin Interactions

Medication is typically a part of your everyday routine while managing a chronic condition like diabetes. Remember, too, that like other medications, metformin can interact with other prescriptions, over-the-counter vitamins, and even specific foods.

These combinations could potentially increase the risk of side effects or impair the effectiveness of metformin. It is possible to make safer and better health-related decisions if you are aware of these possible interactions.

Drug-Drug Interactions

To treat other medical illnesses or to control their diabetes, many patients with Type 2 diabetes take many medications.

Notwithstanding the fact that metformin is usually safe and well-tolerated, it can interact with other drugs in ways that impair kidney function, blood sugar regulation, or pharmaceutical effectiveness.

Certain drugs may increase blood sugar levels, negating the benefits of metformin and making it more difficult to properly control your diabetes. These consist of:

Corticosteroids: Anti-inflammatory medications such as prednisone might increase blood sugar, which reduces the effectiveness of metformin.

Diuretics: Blood sugar regulation may be impacted by diuretics, which aid in the body's removal of surplus water. These drugs may also have an impact on how well your kidneys handle metformin.

Antipsychotic: Blood sugar regulation may be disrupted by certain antipsychotic medications, which are used to treat mental health issues like schizophrenia and bipolar disorder.

Hormonal therapies: In addition to raising blood sugar levels, estrogen and birth control tablets should be closely watched when taken with metformin.

Your doctor may need to change the dosage of your Metformin or suggest more frequent blood sugar checks if you take any of these medications in order to keep your levels steady.

Supplements and Herbal Remedies

Supplements and herbal cures can interact with drugs such as Metformin, despite their common perception as natural and harmless.

Tell your doctor if you take supplements for any other health concerns so they can determine if there could be any interactions.

Vitamin B12: Over time, a possible deficit may result from Metformin's reduction in vitamin B12 absorption. To monitor your levels and modify your dosage if necessary, your doctor might advise routine blood tests if you use a B12 supplement.

Magnesium: Supplementing with magnesium might impact how your body metabolizes metformin and can also cause cramping in your muscles or cardiac problems.

If taking magnesium is safe for you, your health care practitioner can advise you on that.

Ginseng: Research indicates that when used with Metformin, ginseng may drop blood sugar levels and raise the risk of hypoglycemia.

Food Interactions

While most meals can be taken with metformin without issue, the effectiveness of the medicine may be affected by some dietary choices.

You can maintain Metformin's ability to effectively regulate your blood sugar by making minor dietary modifications.

Alcohol: One of the most important interactions with Metformin to be mindful of is alcohol consumption. A rare but dangerous disorder called lactic acidosis, in which lactic acid accumulates in the bloodstream, can be made more likely by binge drinking alcohol.

Alcohol can create harmful levels of lactic acid when coupled with metformin because it alters how your liver processes the acid.

High-Fiber Foods: Consuming a diet high in fiber is good for your health generally, but eating a diet too high in fiber can make it harder for your body to absorb metformin.

Consuming a lot of fiber can possibly lower the amount of Metformin your body absorbs, which can have an impact on blood sugar regulation. Examples of high-fiber meals and supplements that may help with this include beans and whole grains.

It's critical to maintain a healthy digestive tract and blood sugar regulation, therefore it's necessary to balance your consumption of fiber.

However, too much fiber may cause you to change your Metformin dosage. If you're not sure how much fiber is appropriate for you, talk to your health care professional about your diet.

Chapter Eight

Overdose

Anyone taking medicine for a chronic illness like diabetes has to be concerned about the danger of inadvertently taking too much of it.

Taking too much metformin can result in serious consequences, even though it is typically thought to be safe and effective.

A uncommon but potentially fatal condition known as lactic acidosis can arise from a Metformin overdose and necessitates prompt medical intervention.

It can help you to stay safe while treating your diabetes if you know the warning signs of an overdose, how to prevent it, and what to do in an emergency.

When a person takes more medicine than their body can metabolize, it's called an overdose. An overabundance of metformin can cause lactic acidosis, a potentially fatal illness marked by an accumulation of lactic acid in the blood.

Symptoms

A speedy recovery or a major health disaster may depend on your ability to identify the early indicators of a Metformin overdose.

When an overdose occurs, the following symptoms may initially seem similar to typical Metformin adverse effects:

- Nausea
- Vomiting
- Diarrhea
- Weakness or fatigue
- Abdominal discomfort

If these early symptoms develop or persist, they may be a sign of something more serious than the usual side effects related to the digestive system.

Severe Symptoms

With the onset of lactic acidosis, symptoms may worsen and intensify:

- Difficulty breathing or shortness of breath
- Dizziness or lightheadedness
- Rapid or irregular heartbeat
- Extreme tiredness or weakness that doesn't improve with rest
- Extreme muscle pain or cramping
- Feeling unusually cold, especially in the hands and feet

Prompt medical attention is necessary for these symptoms. Seeking immediate medical attention is imperative if you or anyone else exhibits any of these symptoms following a Metformin overdose.

It is imperative to take immediate action if you believe that you or someone else may have taken an excessive amount of metformin. Failure to treat a metformin overdose promptly can be fatal, particularly if it results in lactic acidosis.

It is imperative to take immediate action if you believe that you or someone else may have taken an excessive amount of metformin. Failure to treat a metformin overdose promptly can be fatal, particularly if it results in lactic acidosis.

Prevention

Dial 911 right away if you think someone may have overdosed. Details regarding the metformin dosage used should be included in your thorough explanation of the circumstances.

Seeking prompt medical attention is crucial, even if the symptoms initially appear to be minor. Early treatment is essential because lactic acidosis can progress quickly.

Remain composed and comfort the overdose victim while you wait for medical assistance. Maintain their comfort while keeping an eye on their respiration and level of awareness.

Following your doctor's instructions closely is the best defense against a Metformin overdose.

You can lower your risk of taking too much Metformin, even if mishaps do happen. As directed by your doctor, take Metformin exactly as directed at all times.

If the drug doesn't seem to be functioning as well as it should, don't ever change the dosage on your own. Before making any changes, discuss any worries you may have about your dose with your doctor.

Use a Pill Organizer

An pill organizer can be useful if you take more than one prescription or have trouble remembering when you last took your dose.

It's easier to manage your medication without running the risk of doubling up when you use our easy-to-use tool to plan out your daily doses.

Utilize your phone's alarm or reminder features to assist you in remembering to take your prescription at the same time every day. Because of missing doses, this can stop Metformin from being accidentally overused.

Chapter Nine

Storage

Medication storage practices are equally crucial as dosage methods. Maintaining the efficacy and safety of metformin over time can be achieved by storing it properly.

Adhering to the proper storage standards is crucial to safeguard your health and the health of those you love, even though it may seem like a straightforward undertaking.

Drugs are affected by temperature, humidity, and light, among other surroundings. Some factors have the ability to reduce the efficiency of metformin and jeopardize your health if it is not stored properly.

To guarantee that you obtain the greatest benefit from your therapy, proper storage keeps Metformin potent from the day you receive it until you finish the prescription.

It is possible that metformin will be less effective in controlling your blood sugar levels if it is stored in humid or extremely hot conditions.

Medication stored in an unhygienic environment may introduce moisture or germs that could be harmful to your health.

It can be problematic if children are around and medication is kept in widely accessible places where they could be accidentally consumed.

Your medication will continue to be secure and effective if you store metformin properly, shielding both you and other people from these dangers. At room temperature, which is normally between 68°F and 77°F (20°C and 25°C), metformin should be stored.

Extreme temperature can reduce the medication's effectiveness, so try to keep it away. Metformin's effectiveness is greatly threatened by humidity.

Keep your medication out of the kitchen and bathroom where moisture from cooking and steam from showers can get in.

Rather, select a cool, dry location, like a medicine cabinet that isn't humid or a drawer in your bedroom. Metformin can also deteriorate over time when exposed to strong light or direct sunshine.

It's important to maintain the drug in its original, light-resistant packaging. For an additional degree of security, if the bottle is packaged, think about keeping it in the box.

To stop pollutants, moisture, or air from getting inside, make sure the bottle is tightly closed after every use.

Safe Storage Around Children and Pets

To avoid accidental intake, which poses major health hazards, including overdose, it is imperative to keep medication out of the reach of children and dogs. The best place to keep metformin is somewhere out of reach for paws or hands that could get intrigued.

Metformin should be kept in a high cabinet, ideally one with a lock, if you have children or pets at home.

As a result, children and animals cannot inadvertently consume the drug. To keep kids from opening the bottle, most Metformin bottles come with a child-resistant cap.

Make sure the cap is firmly fastened after each use and always store the medication in its original package. It is important to educate older kids about the risks associated with taking over-the-counter medications.

Inform them that taking Metformin or any other drug should never be done so without a doctor's supervision and that it is exclusively for the individual to whom it is prescribed.

Keeping your medication secure and shielding your family from potential danger are two benefits of taking these extra precautions.

Metformin while traveling

The proper way to keep Metformin when traveling should be taken into consideration. Maintaining the effectiveness of your prescription while traveling guarantees that it will follow you wherever life leads you, whether you're traveling locally or across the globe.

Always carry on your luggage when traveling by air, never check in. This includes your Metformin. Excessive temperatures in the cargo hold may be experienced by checked baggage, potentially compromising the effectiveness of the prescription.

It guarantees that you will have access to it in the event of delays or misplaced luggage if you pack it in your carry-on.

Disposal and Expiration

It's important to be aware of the expiration date of any drug. Your health may be at risk if you take expired Metformin since it may become less effective.

It is in your and your family's best interests to know when and how to properly dispose of outdated medications. Usually printed on the bottle or package is the expiration date of metformin.

It is imperative that you routinely verify this date, particularly if your prescription is almost finished. In order to avoid medication not working as intended, do not take Metformin after its expiration date.

How to Dispose of Expired Metformin

You must properly dispose of the previous prescription when your Metformin runs out or if your doctor wants to switch up your dosage. Metformin shouldn't be disposed of or flushed down the toilet because doing so could harm the ecosystem. Instead:

For unneeded or expired pharmaceuticals, many pharmacies have take-back schemes in place. To find out if your neighborhood drugstore participates, ask them.

The FDA suggests sealing the medication in a plastic bag, tossing it in the household garbage, and combining it with an unattractive item, like used coffee grounds or cat litter, if a take-back program isn't offered. This decreases the possibility of someone swallowing the drug by accident.

The End